Sciatica: What a pain in the A***!

An in-depth guide not the management, treatment and prevention of sciatic

By Arun Gray BSc

Contents

Heading
Introduction
Understanding Sciatica
What is Sciatica?
Causes of Sciatica
Diagnosing Sciatica
Managing Sciatica Pain
Understanding Pain
Immediate Pain Relief Strategies
The Role of Exercise
Treating Sciatica
Non-Surgical Treatments
When Surgery is Necessary
Preventing Sciatica
Building a Resilient Body
Ergonomics & Lifestyle Changes
Long Term Strategies
Resources and Support
Frequently Asked Questions
Tools and Resources
When to Seek Help
Closing Thoughts

Introduction

My name's Arun Gray. I'm a sports therapist and strength and conditioning coach with over a decade of experience working in gyms, professional sport and private sports injury clinics.

This is my second book. In my first one (What the ACL F**k?) I explain my personal history with ACL injuries… now I'm going to sound like I'm made of glass here, but I've got my fair share of memories of sciatica, too!

It all really started when I did what most lads in their early 20's do when they go to the gym… I tried to lift a weight that I really wasn't strong enough to lift properly.

I suffered a herniated disc which essentially put pressure on my sciatic nerve and left me with some pretty brutal electric-shock-like pains down my leg.

This isn't always the cause of sciatic nerve pain, which I'll explain later in the book. But it is a common one. If you've seen any of my back pain related TikTok's, you might have heard me preach about how you can't slip a disc and you also can't trap a nerve… A herniated disc pressing on the nerve however, is usually what people are describing. So a little later on I'll explain the anatomy of these and how it causes that dreaded sciatica pain. This will hopefully help you understand what's going on with your body, how you can manage it and ideally stop it coming back in the future.

Why I wrote this book?

I wrote this book for two main reasons. The first one is that over the last 8 years of me doing this job, sciatica and lower back pain are the most common presenting 'injury' in my clinics, by some distance. Which I can only imagine means it's something quite common in the general public.

Unless by some strange coincidence Lincolnshire has an absurdly high rate of sciatica across the county... However back in lock down when I started sharing TikToks on various injuries and painful conditions, a video on how to test if you have sciatica at home was my first viral video, getting millions of views and leading to me being interviewed for the LadBible.

Which again, I can only assume was because it resonated with so many people!

The second, and the one that really grinds my gears, is that there is so much misinformation online when it comes to sciatica. When writing this book, it didn't take me long to find the NHS still referring to people "slipping their discs" on **their website**. Can you believe that?! You can't slip a disc... it's physically impossible. And yes, it might be a way of GP's and medical professionals speaking in language that people understand, but it's scientifically and anatomically inaccurate... so why they're still using those terms really does royally p**s me off!

You probably don't think it's that much of a big deal. Which is fair. But it makes people think they are "unfixable" and leads them to thinking they have a bad back forever, which simply isn't true.

Sure, there are some people who unfortunately have to live with chronic back pain and there isn't much they can do. But for the general population, there are things you can do to improve your symptoms.

Anyway, you've got me ranting.

I wrote the book to show people there is things you can do, you're not broken, and I'll explain why… without using outdated scare-mongering terms.

Who is this book for?

I'm biased (obviously) but everyone. I guess those most in need are those who tick one of the following boxes:

- ☐ You have sciatica

- ☐ You often/sometimes get sciatica

- ☐ You work with people who suffer from sciatica

- ☐ You want to learn more about sciatica to prevent getting it

If you tick any of those boxes, you've made the right decision by ordering this book.

If you haven't… don't rush to send it back for a refund!!

Around half of the population suffer from back pain and/or sciatica at some point in their lives. In theory, if every single person on the planet read and implemented the information in this book - I'd be a **rich** bloke.

Joking (kind of).

But seriously, if you do read this book and understand it, you'll understand the causes of sciatica and how to prevent it. Now not all cases are preventable (pregnancy, car accidents, sports injuries) but a lot of the generic day-to-day cases are.

So having the information in this book in your head will put you in a good place to staying healthy and pain free. Think of it as the answer a really specific pub quiz question. You might not ever need to know if, but if you do… bosh.

How to use this book?

It's written to be used as a reference. Buying it off Amazon won't fix your back pain. But reading it should hopefully help you understand what's causing your pain. And if you can understand the cause, you are a huge step closer to finding a way of managing your symptoms.

Part 1: Understanding Sciatica

Chapter 1: What is sciatica?

In this chapter, I'll go through an introduction into the condition. I'll give you a definition of what sciatica is and explain the causes of the pain itself. I'll talk you through the signs and symptoms (which you might have already felt for yourself!) So that you know how to recognise some of the symptoms if you or a friend/relative are suffering with it.

Then I'll take you through some of the myths and misconceptions that commonly get circulated about sciatica. It's a common 'injury' so there's plenty to choose from.

I'll give you a quick one to start…. You **cannot** (and I can't emphasise that enough) slip a disc.

I'll leave that there for now.

What is "Sciatica"?

Sciatica is a term that many people have heard, but few truly understand. It is often mistakenly used to describe any lower back pain, but in reality, sciatica is a specific type of nerve pain that radiates along the path of the sciatic nerve. This nerve, the longest in the human body, runs from the lower back, through the hips and buttocks, and down each leg. When something irritates or compresses the sciatic nerve, it can lead to a range of painful symptoms that affect daily life.

Sciatica is usually caused by compression or irritation of the sciatic nerve, which can result from a variety of conditions. The most common cause is a herniated or bulging (often inaccurately referred to as "slipped") disc in the lower spine, which presses against the nerve and leads to pain and discomfort.

Other causes include spinal stenosis, which is a narrowing of the spinal canal; degenerative disc disease, where the discs between vertebrae deteriorate over time; and piriformis syndrome, where the piriformis muscle in the buttock becomes inflamed and irritates the sciatic nerve. Additionally, lifestyle factors such as prolonged sitting, poor posture, or repetitive movements that strain the lower back can contribute to the development of sciatica.

Sciatica signs and symptoms

The symptoms of sciatica can vary in intensity, but they typically include pain that starts in the lower back or buttock and travels down the back of the leg. This pain can be sharp, shooting, or burning, and it may be accompanied by tingling, numbness, or muscle weakness in the affected leg. Some people describe the sensation as an electric shock running down their leg, while others experience a dull, persistent ache. In more severe cases, sciatica can make it difficult to stand, walk, or even sit comfortably for extended periods.

The severity of sciatica symptoms often depends on the underlying cause. For example, a herniated disc pressing directly on the nerve root may cause intense pain, while a mild irritation from muscle tightness may produce a more manageable level of discomfort. However it's important to note that the level of pain isn't enough to provide you with a diagnosis of the cause. More pain doesn't necessarily mean a worse condition.

Some people find that their symptoms worsen after long periods of sitting or standing, while others struggle with pain first thing in the morning. Sciatica can also lead to difficulty in performing everyday activities, such as bending down to tie a shoe or climbing stairs.

Myths and Misconceptions

Despite how common sciatica is, there are many myths and misconceptions surrounding it. One of the biggest misconceptions is that sciatica is a condition in itself, rather than a symptom of an underlying issue. Sciatica is usually caused by something pressing on or irritating the sciatic nerve, such as a herniated disc, spinal stenosis, or even tight muscles like the piriformis. Another myth is that sciatica always requires surgery. While surgery can be necessary in extreme cases, the vast majority of people with sciatica can manage and even resolve their symptoms through conservative treatments such as physiotherapy, targeted exercises, and lifestyle adjustments.

Another common misconception is that bed rest is the best solution for sciatica. While it may seem logical to rest when in pain, prolonged inactivity can actually make symptoms worse. Movement and gentle stretching often play a crucial role in recovery. Similarly, many people believe that sciatica only affects older adults, but it can develop at any age, particularly in those who perform repetitive movements, sit for long periods, or engage in activities that put strain on the lower back.

Some people also believe that sciatica will go away on its own and does not require treatment. While mild cases of sciatica may improve with time, ignoring the symptoms can lead to chronic pain or worsening of the underlying issue. Seeking appropriate treatment, whether through a medical professional, physiotherapy, or self-care techniques, can significantly improve recovery outcomes and prevent future episodes.

Understanding what sciatica truly is, along with its symptoms and the myths surrounding it, is the first step toward managing it effectively. By gaining a clearer picture of how sciatica develops and how it affects the body, individuals can take proactive steps to address their pain and improve their quality of life. With the right approach, it is possible to reduce symptoms, enhance mobility, and return to normal activities with greater ease.

Chapter 2: Causes of Sciatica

In this short chapter, I'll discuss what commonly causes sciatica. Knowing this helps you both treat and prevent commonly caused sciatica pain.

I'll discuss common injuries such as herniated discs which irritative or compress the nerve, causing pain as well as other potential causes; before discussing lifestyle factors that usually trigger the underlying injuries, before finally touching on the more severe things to look out for and when you might need a trip to the hospital.

The Sciatic Nerve and it's Roles

The sciatic nerve is the largest and longest nerve in the human body, extending from the lower back down through the hips, buttocks, and legs. It plays a crucial role in transmitting signals between the spinal cord and the lower limbs, allowing for movement and sensation. This nerve is responsible for enabling functions such as walking, running, and even standing, making it essential to overall mobility. When the sciatic nerve becomes irritated or compressed, it can lead to sciatica, a condition characterised by pain and discomfort along its pathway.

Underlying Injuries

There are several structural causes of sciatica, with herniated discs being one of the most common. A herniated disc occurs when the soft inner portion of a spinal disc pushes through the tough outer layer, placing pressure on nearby nerves, including the sciatic nerve. This compression can lead to inflammation, pain, and neurological symptoms such as tingling or numbness in the legs. Spinal stenosis is another structural cause, occurring when the spinal canal narrows and compresses the nerves. This is often a result of age-related changes, such as thickened ligaments or bone spurs, which reduce the available space for the nerves. Other structural causes include degenerative disc disease, spondylolisthesis (a condition where one vertebra slips over another), and sacroiliac joint dysfunction, all of which can contribute to sciatic nerve irritation.

Lifestyle and Occupational Factors

Lifestyle and occupational factors can also play a significant role in the development of sciatica. Prolonged sitting, particularly with poor posture, can place excessive strain on the lower back and contribute to nerve compression. Jobs that require heavy lifting, twisting, or repetitive movements can also increase the risk of developing sciatica. Additionally, obesity places extra stress on the spine, which can exacerbate existing spinal conditions and contribute to sciatic nerve irritation. Even seemingly harmless daily habits, such as carrying a wallet in the back pocket while sitting, can contribute to sciatic discomfort by putting pressure on the nerve over time.

Red Flags & Emergencies

While structural and lifestyle factors are common causes of sciatica, there are also rarer causes that should not be overlooked. Tumours growing near the spine can exert pressure on the sciatic nerve, leading to severe pain and other neurological symptoms. Infections affecting the spine, such as abscesses or osteomyelitis, can also lead to sciatic nerve compression. Another rare but serious cause is cauda equina syndrome, a condition that results from severe nerve compression and requires immediate medical attention. Symptoms of this syndrome include loss of bladder or bowel control, severe weakness in the legs, and numbness in the saddle area (inner thighs and buttocks). These red flags indicate a medical emergency that requires prompt intervention to prevent permanent nerve damage.

Understanding the various causes of sciatica can help individuals identify risk factors and take proactive measures to prevent or manage their condition. Whether sciatica is caused by structural issues, lifestyle choices, or rare medical conditions, addressing the underlying cause is essential for effective treatment and long-term relief.

Chapter 3: Diagnosing Sciatica

In this final chapter of part 1, I'll explain how a medical professional goes about diagnosing sciatica; the first step in finding a way to treat it. As I explained earlier, 'sciatica' is more of a symptom than an injury itself. It's usually caused by another underlying injury or muscle skeletal problem which isn't agreeing with the nerve. So finding and treating that is key to getting you back on your (pain-free) feet.

Diagnoses by Healthcare Professionals

Diagnosing sciatica requires a thorough evaluation by a healthcare professional, as the symptoms can sometimes overlap with other conditions affecting the lower back and legs. The diagnostic process typically begins with a detailed medical history and physical examination. A doctor will ask about the onset of symptoms, their severity, and any activities that worsen or relieve the pain. They may also inquire about past injuries, medical conditions, and lifestyle factors that could contribute to sciatic nerve irritation.

During the physical examination, a healthcare provider may perform a series of tests to assess nerve function, muscle strength, and range of motion. One common test is the straight leg raise test, in which the patient lies on their back while the doctor gently lifts one leg. If this movement triggers pain radiating down the leg, it may indicate sciatica. Other clinical assessments, such as checking reflexes and sensation in the lower limbs, help to determine the extent of nerve involvement.

Imaging and Tests

In some cases, additional imaging tests are necessary to confirm the diagnosis and identify the underlying cause of sciatica. X-rays can reveal spinal abnormalities such as bone spurs or fractures that may be compressing the sciatic nerve.

Magnetic resonance imaging (MRI) is often the preferred method for visualising soft tissues, including herniated discs and nerve impingements. Computed tomography (CT) scans with myelography can provide detailed images of the spinal canal, particularly in cases of suspected spinal stenosis. Electromyography (EMG) and nerve conduction studies may be used to assess nerve function and identify any nerve damage.

Not everyone with sciatica requires imaging tests, as the majority of cases can be diagnosed based on symptoms and physical examination alone. However, imaging may be recommended if symptoms persist for more than six weeks, are severe, or if there are signs of serious conditions such as tumours, infections, or cauda equina syndrome.

Self-Assessment Tools

For those experiencing sciatic pain, self-assessment tools can help determine whether professional evaluation is necessary. Keeping a pain diary that tracks the location, intensity, and duration of symptoms can be useful in identifying patterns and triggers. Simple movement tests, such as the straight leg raise performed at home, can also indicate potential sciatic nerve involvement. However, self-assessment should never replace professional medical advice, especially if symptoms worsen or include red flags such as significant weakness, loss of bowel or bladder control, or unrelenting pain.

Understanding how sciatica is diagnosed can give people the nudge to seek timely medical attention and take proactive steps toward effective treatment. Whether through clinical evaluation, imaging investigation, or self-awareness, a proper diagnosis is the first step in managing and overcoming sciatic pain.

Part 2: Managing Sciatica Pain

Chapter 4: Understanding Pain

Pain is more than just a physical sensation—it's a complex experience shaped by the nervous system and the brain. Sciatica, a condition caused by irritation or compression of the sciatic nerve, produces pain that is often described as sharp, burning, or electric-like. Unlike pain from muscles or joints, this type of nerve pain originates from dysfunction within the nervous system, making it particularly difficult to ignore.

In this chapter, I'll explain what makes sciatica pain unique, the differences between acute and chronic pain, and how the brain plays a critical role in pain perception. Chronic sciatica, in particular, can persist even after the original injury has healed, sometimes due to an overactive nervous system amplifying pain signals. Emotional and psychological factors, such as stress and anxiety, can also heighten pain levels, creating a frustrating cycle for sufferers.

By understanding the science behind why sciatica hurts, we can take a more informed and proactive approach to pain management. From physical treatments to strategies that retrain the brain's response to pain, this chapter lays the groundwork for overcoming sciatica and reclaiming control over your well-being.

Why sciatica hurts: The science of nerve pain

Pain is one of the most complex experiences of the human body, and sciatica-related pain is no exception. Understanding why sciatica hurts requires a look at the science of nerve pain. The sciatic nerve is the largest in the body, running from the lower back down through the buttocks and legs. When this nerve becomes irritated or compressed, it sends pain signals to the brain, which are often described as sharp, burning, or electric-like sensations. This is because nerve pain, or neuropathic pain, differs from musculoskeletal pain, which usually stems from muscle or joint issues. Instead of originating from tissue damage alone, neuropathic pain is caused by dysfunction within the nervous system itself, making it particularly difficult to ignore.

The difference between acute and chronic pain

There is also an important distinction between acute and chronic pain when it comes to sciatica. Acute pain is short-term, typically lasting less than three months, and usually resolves as the underlying cause heals. For instance, if a herniated disc is the culprit, sciatica pain may subside once the disc is reabsorbed or inflammation decreases. Chronic pain, however, persists beyond this timeframe and may continue even after the initial injury has healed. This can occur due to prolonged nerve irritation, nerve damage, or changes in how the nervous system processes pain signals. Chronic sciatica can be particularly frustrating because the brain may become overly sensitised, amplifying pain responses even when the original cause is no longer present.

The role of the brain and emotions in pain

The brain plays a crucial role in how pain is perceived and experienced. Pain is not just a direct result of physical damage; it is also influenced by emotions, stress, and psychological factors. The brain interprets pain signals based on past experiences, expectations, and even mood. This means that anxiety, depression, and high levels of stress can actually make sciatica pain feel worse. When the nervous system remains in a heightened state of alertness, it can lead to a cycle where pain persists even in the absence of an ongoing physical problem.

Understanding the relationship between the brain and pain has led to advancements in pain management strategies. Techniques such as mindfulness, cognitive behavioural therapy, and relaxation exercises can help retrain the brain's response to pain. This does not mean that sciatica pain is imagined or purely psychological, but rather that managing emotional and mental well-being can have a significant impact on pain levels. Combining these approaches with physical treatment, such as physiotherapy or targeted exercises, can lead to better overall outcomes for individuals suffering from sciatica.

By gaining a deeper understanding of why sciatica hurts, the differences between acute and chronic pain, and the role the brain plays in pain perception, individuals can take a more informed and proactive approach to managing their symptoms. Recognising that pain is influenced by multiple factors opens the door to more comprehensive treatment strategies, ultimately helping people regain control over their condition and improve their quality of life.

Chapter 5: Immediate Pain Relief Strategies

When sciatica pain strikes, finding immediate relief is often a top priority. While long-term strategies are essential for preventing recurrence, there are several effective methods for quickly managing pain in the moment. Understanding and using these strategies correctly can make a significant difference in reducing discomfort and improving mobility.

Safe and Effective Stretches

Stretching is one of the most effective ways to relieve sciatic pain. By reducing tension in the muscles surrounding the sciatic nerve, stretching can alleviate pressure and improve flexibility. However, it's crucial to perform these stretches correctly to avoid exacerbating symptoms.

One highly effective stretch is the piriformis stretch, which targets a small muscle deep in the buttocks that can contribute to sciatic nerve compression. To perform this stretch, sit on the floor with one leg bent and the other crossed over it, placing the foot flat on the ground. Gently twist your torso toward the bent knee, holding the stretch for 20-30 seconds before switching sides.

Another beneficial stretch is the seated spinal twist, which helps improve spinal mobility and reduce nerve irritation. Sitting on a chair with both feet flat on the ground, twist your upper body to one side, holding the armrest or back of the chair for support. Hold for 20-30 seconds and repeat on the opposite side.

The hamstring stretch can also provide relief, as tight hamstrings can increase tension on the lower back. Lying on your back, lift one leg while keeping it straight and gently pull it toward you using a towel or resistance band. Hold for 20-30 seconds and switch sides.

Heat vs. Ice: When and How to Use Them

Both heat and ice therapy can help manage sciatic pain, but they serve different purposes. Knowing when to use each method can make a big difference in symptom relief.

Ice therapy (cryotherapy) is most effective in the early stages of a sciatic flare-up. Cold packs help reduce inflammation and numb sharp pain. Apply an ice pack wrapped in a towel to the lower back or affected area for 15-20 minutes at a time, several times a day. Avoid direct skin contact to prevent frostbite.

Heat therapy is more beneficial for muscle tightness and chronic pain. Applying a heating pad or warm compress to the lower back can improve blood flow, relax tight muscles, and ease discomfort. Use heat therapy for 20-30 minutes as needed, but avoid excessive heat exposure to prevent burns.

For some individuals, alternating between heat and ice, known as contrast therapy, can be particularly effective. Using ice first to reduce inflammation, followed by heat to relax the muscles, can provide the best of both treatments.

Over-the-Counter Medications: Pros and Cons

For those experiencing significant pain, over-the-counter (OTC) medications can provide temporary relief. However, it's important to understand the benefits and limitations of each type.

Nonsteroidal anti-inflammatory drugs (NSAIDs) like ibuprofen and naproxen help reduce inflammation and alleviate pain. These medications can be effective for short-term relief but should not be used for extended periods without consulting a healthcare professional, as they can cause stomach irritation and other side effects.

Acetaminophen (paracetamol) is another common pain reliever that works by altering the brain's perception of pain. While it does not reduce inflammation, it can be a suitable alternative for individuals who cannot take NSAIDs.

Topical pain relief creams containing ingredients like menthol, capsaicin, or lidocaine can also provide localised relief by numbing the affected area and reducing discomfort.

While OTC medications can be helpful, they should be used as part of a broader treatment plan rather than a long-term solution. Persistent or worsening symptoms should always be evaluated by a healthcare provider.

Alternative Remedies: Acupuncture, Massage, and More

In addition to traditional pain relief methods, alternative therapies can play a role in managing sciatic pain. Many individuals find relief through practices that focus on relaxation, circulation, and nerve function.

Acupuncture, a technique rooted in traditional Chinese medicine, involves inserting thin needles into specific points on the body to promote pain relief and healing. Research suggests that acupuncture can help reduce nerve pain by stimulating endorphin release and improving blood flow to the affected area.

Massage therapy can also be beneficial, particularly deep tissue or trigger point massage, which targets muscle knots and tension that may be contributing to sciatic pain. A skilled massage therapist can focus on the lower back, glutes, and hamstrings to release pressure on the sciatic nerve.

Chiropractic adjustments may help reestablish spinal mobility and reduce nerve compression. Many individuals with sciatica report improvement after spinal manipulation, although the effectiveness of this treatment varies from person to person.

Yoga and Pilates incorporate gentle movements and stretches that promote flexibility and core strength, both of which are essential for reducing sciatic pain and preventing future flare-ups.

Immediate pain relief strategies can provide much-needed comfort during sciatic flare-ups, but they work best when combined with a long-term approach to treatment. By using a mix of stretching, heat and ice therapy, over the counter medications, and alternative remedies, individuals can manage their symptoms effectively while addressing the root causes of their pain. Consulting with a healthcare provider before beginning any treatment plan ensures that relief methods are safe and appropriate for each individual's condition.

Chapter 6: The Role of Exercise

When dealing with sciatica, the instinct may be to rest and avoid movement, but staying active is one of the most effective ways to reduce pain and support recovery. Movement plays a crucial role in maintaining flexibility, strengthening the muscles that support the spine, and improving circulation—all of which help alleviate pressure on the sciatic nerve and promote healing. In contrast, prolonged rest can lead to stiffness, muscle weakening, and worsening symptoms over time.

In this chapter, I discuss why movement is essential for sciatica recovery, starting with gentle stretches and mobility exercises that relieve tension around the sciatic nerve. We then discuss the importance of core strengthening to stabilise the spine, followed by low-impact activities like walking and swimming that promote long-term spinal health. Knowing how to progress safely and when to modify exercises ensures that people can stay active without aggravating their condition.

Why movement is essential for recovery

Exercise plays a crucial role in the recovery process for individuals suffering from sciatica. While it may seem counterintuitive to move when in pain, staying active is one of the most effective ways to reduce discomfort and prevent future flare-ups. Movement helps maintain flexibility, strengthens the muscles that support the spine, and improves circulation, all of which contribute to better overall spinal health. Prolonged rest, on the other hand, can lead to stiffness, muscle weakening, and increased pain over time.

One of the key benefits of exercise for sciatica is its ability to relieve pressure on the sciatic nerve. Gentle movements help reduce inflammation and promote healing by encouraging blood flow to the affected area. Additionally, maintaining mobility helps prevent compensatory movement patterns that can lead to further discomfort. The key is to start with low-impact exercises that do not put excessive strain on the lower back or aggravate the nerve.

Gentle exercises to start with

When beginning an exercise routine for sciatica relief, gentle stretching and mobility exercises should be the first step. These exercises aim to improve flexibility in the lower back, hips, and legs while relieving tension around the sciatic nerve. A simple knee-to-chest stretch can be a good starting point. Lying on the back, one knee is gently pulled toward the chest while keeping the other leg straight, holding the position for 20-30 seconds before switching sides. Another effective movement is the cat-cow stretch, which involves alternating between arching and rounding the back while on hands and knees, promoting spinal mobility and reducing stiffness.

Progression to strengthening and core stability

Once initial mobility and flexibility have improved, the next step is to incorporate strengthening exercises that support the lower back and core. Weak core muscles can contribute to poor posture and spinal instability, which can exacerbate sciatic pain. Engaging in gentle core exercises, such as pelvic tilts and bridges, helps develop strength in the muscles surrounding the spine. For instance, performing a bridge exercise by lying on the back with knees bent and lifting the hips toward the ceiling strengthens the lower back and gluteal muscles, providing additional support to the spine.

As strength and flexibility improve, progressing to more dynamic movements can further enhance spinal stability and overall function. Exercises such as bird-dogs and modified planks help build endurance in the core without putting excessive stress on the lower back. The bird-dog exercise involves extending one arm and the opposite leg while on hands and knees, holding the position briefly before switching sides. This movement promotes balance and coordination while engaging key stabilizing muscles.

Gradually incorporating aerobic activities such as walking or swimming can also be beneficial for overall spinal health. These low-impact exercises help maintain cardiovascular fitness, improve circulation, and support weight management, all of which contribute to reducing strain on the lower back. Walking, in particular, encourages natural spinal movement and helps prevent stiffness, making it an excellent addition to a sciatica exercise routine.

While exercise is essential for recovery, it is important to listen to the body and avoid movements that cause sharp or worsening pain. Individuals should progress at their own pace and consult a healthcare professional or physical therapist to ensure they are following a safe and effective program. By incorporating regular movement, gentle stretching, and progressive strengthening, individuals can regain mobility, reduce pain, and build resilience against future sciatic issues.

Part 3: Treating Sciatica

Chapter 7: Non-surgical treatments

When dealing with sciatica, the natural instinct might be to rest and avoid movement—but staying active is actually one of the most effective ways to reduce pain and aid recovery. Movement keeps the spine flexible, strengthens the muscles that support it, and improves circulation, all of which help relieve pressure on the sciatic nerve and promote healing. In contrast, prolonged inactivity can lead to stiffness, muscle weakness, and worsening pain over time.

This chapter explores why movement is a crucial part of sciatica recovery and how specific exercises can help. We begin with gentle stretching and mobility movements designed to ease tension around the sciatic nerve before progressing to core-strengthening exercises that provide stability and support for the lower back. As strength improves, incorporating low-impact activities like walking or swimming can further enhance recovery while reducing the risk of future flare-ups.

The key to successful recovery is finding the right balance—moving regularly without overloading the body. By understanding the role of movement and following a structured progression, individuals can regain mobility, reduce discomfort, and build long-term resilience against sciatic pain.

For many individuals suffering from sciatica, non-surgical treatments provide an effective means of managing pain and improving function without the need for invasive procedures. A variety of approaches, including physiotherapy, chiropractic care, and targeted pain management techniques, can help reduce discomfort and support long-term recovery. Understanding these options allows individuals to make informed decisions about their treatment plan and find the best approach for their specific condition.

Physiotherapy: What to expect and how it helps

Physiotherapy: What to expect and how it helpsPhysiotherapy is one of the most recommended treatments for sciatica, as it focuses on restoring mobility, strengthening the supporting muscles, and preventing future episodes of pain. A physiotherapist will typically begin with a thorough assessment to identify the underlying causes of sciatic nerve irritation. Treatment often includes a combination of stretching exercises, strength-building movements, and manual therapy techniques. Stretching exercises help improve flexibility in the lower back, hips, and legs, relieving pressure on the sciatic nerve. Strength-building movements target the core and lower back muscles, improving spinal stability and reducing the risk of recurring pain. Manual therapy, which may include techniques such as massage and joint mobilisation, helps reduce muscle tightness and improve spinal alignment. Patients undergoing physiotherapy will also receive guidance on posture correction and movement modifications to minimise strain on the lower back during daily activities.

Chiropractic care: Does it work?

Another common non-surgical treatment for sciatica is chiropractic care, which focuses on spinal alignment and nerve function. Chiropractors use spinal adjustments and manipulations to relieve pressure on the sciatic nerve, improving mobility and reducing pain. Many individuals report experiencing relief from chiropractic treatments, particularly when sciatica is caused by misaligned vertebrae or joint dysfunction. However, chiropractic care is not suitable for all cases of sciatica, particularly if the underlying cause involves conditions such as severe disc herniation or spinal stenosis. It is essential to consult with a healthcare professional before pursuing chiropractic treatment to determine if it is an appropriate option.

Pain management techniques

Pain management techniques can also be valuable in reducing sciatic discomfort, particularly for those experiencing severe or persistent symptoms. One common approach is the use of

Transcutaneous Electrical Nerve Stimulation (TENS) machines. These devices deliver mild electrical impulses to the affected area, disrupting pain signals and promoting muscle relaxation. Many individuals find that using a TENS machine provides temporary relief and can be used alongside other treatments to manage symptoms more effectively.

For individuals with more intense or prolonged sciatic pain, medical professionals may recommend corticosteroid injections. These injections deliver powerful anti-inflammatory medication directly to the affected nerve, reducing swelling and alleviating pain. While corticosteroid injections can provide significant relief, their effects are usually temporary, lasting weeks or months. They are often used as part of a broader treatment plan, rather than as a standalone solution.

Other pain management techniques include acupuncture, which involves inserting thin needles into specific points on the body to stimulate pain relief, and therapeutic massage, which helps relieve muscle tension and improve circulation. Both methods can be effective in reducing sciatic discomfort, though results may vary depending on the individual and the severity of their condition.

Non-surgical treatments offer a wide range of options for managing sciatica, and many individuals find success through a combination of these approaches. By exploring physiotherapy, chiropractic care, and targeted pain management techniques, individuals can develop a comprehensive treatment plan tailored to their needs. Consistency and patience are key, as long-term improvement often requires a multi-faceted approach and ongoing self-care. Consulting with a healthcare professional can help ensure that the chosen treatments are safe, effective, and suitable for each individual's specific condition.

Scan the following QR code for a list of my recommended tools to relieve the symptoms of sciatica:

Chapter 8: When surgery is necessary

While most cases of sciatica improve with non-surgical treatments, there are situations where surgery becomes the best or only option. When symptoms are severe, persistent, or leading to serious complications like loss of bladder or bowel control, surgical intervention may be necessary to relieve pressure on the sciatic nerve and restore function.

This chapter explores the different surgical procedures available, including discectomy, laminectomy, and spinal fusion —each designed to address specific causes of nerve compression. I'll also examine the potential risks and benefits of surgery, helping individuals weigh the likelihood of pain relief against possible complications. Finally, we'll cover what to expect during recovery and rehabilitation, including the role of physical therapy in regaining strength and mobility.

Understanding the surgical process empowers people to make informed decisions about their treatment. While surgery is not always required, for those with debilitating symptoms, it can offer a path to lasting relief and a return to an active life.

While non-surgical treatments can often provide significant relief for sciatica, there are cases where surgery becomes necessary. When symptoms are severe, persistent, or causing serious complications such as loss of bladder or bowel control, surgical intervention may be the best option. Understanding the types of surgeries available, their risks and benefits, and what to expect during recovery can help individuals make informed decisions about their treatment.

Types of surgeries for sciatica

There are several types of surgeries commonly performed to relieve sciatic nerve compression. One of the most frequently used procedures is a discectomy, which involves the removal of a portion of a herniated disc that is pressing on the nerve. This surgery is often recommended when a disc herniation is the primary cause of sciatica and has not responded to conservative treatments. Another option is a laminectomy, which involves the removal of a part of the vertebra called the lamina to create more space for the nerve roots. This procedure is typically performed in cases of spinal stenosis, where the narrowing of the spinal canal compresses the sciatic nerve.

In some cases, spinal fusion may be recommended, particularly if there is instability in the spine due to degenerative conditions or spondylolisthesis. This procedure involves joining two or more vertebrae together using bone grafts and hardware to stabilise the spine. While spinal fusion can provide long-term relief, it also reduces spinal flexibility and may require a longer recovery period.

Risks and benefits

Like any surgical procedure, surgery for sciatica comes with risks and benefits. The primary benefit is the potential for significant pain relief and improved function, particularly for individuals who have not responded to conservative treatments. Many patients experience a substantial reduction in pain and an improvement in mobility within weeks of surgery. However, there are also risks to consider, including infection, nerve damage, blood clots, and complications related to anaesthesia. Additionally, while surgery can address the immediate cause of nerve compression, it does not prevent future spinal issues, and some individuals may still experience recurring symptoms over time.

Recovery and rehabilitation after surgery

Recovery and rehabilitation after surgery play a crucial role in achieving the best possible outcome. Most patients require a period of rest followed by a gradual reintroduction of movement. Physical therapy is often recommended to help regain strength, flexibility, and stability. Early post-operative care typically involves gentle movements, walking, and avoiding heavy lifting or prolonged sitting. As recovery progresses, targeted exercises can help strengthen the core and lower back muscles to reduce the risk of future problems. Full recovery times vary depending on the type of surgery performed, but most individuals can return to normal activities within a few months.

Ultimately, deciding whether to undergo surgery for sciatica is a personal choice that should be made in consultation with a healthcare professional. By weighing the potential benefits against the risks and understanding the recovery process, individuals can make informed decisions about whether surgical intervention is the right path for them. While surgery is not always necessary, for those with severe or disabling symptoms, it can be a life-changing solution that restores quality of life and mobility.

Part 4: Preventing Sciatica

Chapter 9: Building a resilient body

Preventing sciatic pain isn't just about managing symptoms—it's about building a body that is strong, flexible, and resilient against future flare-ups. By strengthening key muscle groups, improving flexibility, and enhancing balance, individuals can create a more stable foundation for spinal health and nerve function.

This chapter explores the essential components of resilience, starting with core and lower body strength to support the spine and reduce strain on the sciatic nerve. We'll also discuss the role of flexibility in keeping muscles pliable and preventing tightness that can contribute to nerve irritation. Finally, we'll cover the importance of balance training to improve coordination, reduce injury risk, and promote better movement patterns.

By incorporating these strategies into a regular routine, individuals can develop a body that is not only more resistant to sciatic pain but also better equipped for daily activities and long-term spinal health.

Building a resilient body is essential for preventing sciatic pain and reducing the likelihood of future flare-ups. Strengthening key muscle groups, improving flexibility, and maintaining good balance all contribute to spinal health and nerve function. By focusing on these aspects, individuals can develop a body that is more resistant to strain and better equipped to handle daily movements and physical activities.

Strengthening key muscle groups

Strengthening the muscles that support the spine is one of the most effective ways to protect against sciatic nerve irritation. The core, which includes the abdominal, oblique, and lower back muscles, plays a crucial role in stabilizing the spine and reducing pressure on the lower back. Weak core muscles can lead to poor posture and increased spinal stress, making sciatica symptoms more likely to occur. Simple exercises such as planks, pelvic tilts, and bird-dogs help engage and strengthen the core without placing excessive strain on the lower back. Additionally, strengthening the gluteal muscles and hamstrings is important for supporting the pelvis and lower spine. Exercises such as squats, hip bridges, and lunges can enhance stability and reduce the likelihood of imbalances that contribute to nerve compression.

Flexibility is equally important for maintaining spinal health and preventing sciatic pain. Tight muscles in the lower back, hips, and legs can contribute to restricted movement and increased tension on the sciatic nerve. Stretching helps keep muscles pliable and reduces the risk of stiffness and strain. Key stretches for sciatica prevention include the piriformis stretch, hamstring stretch, and seated spinal twist. These movements help alleviate tightness in the lower body and promote better mobility. Regular stretching also improves circulation, which aids in muscle recovery and reduces inflammation that can irritate the sciatic nerve.

The importance of flexibility and balance

Balance training is another crucial component of building a resilient body. Poor balance can lead to improper movement patterns, which may contribute to spinal misalignment and increased pressure on the sciatic nerve. Strengthening stabilizing muscles through exercises such as single-leg stands, heel-to-toe walking, and stability ball movements can enhance coordination and reduce the risk of falls or sudden movements that might aggravate sciatica. Engaging in activities such as yoga or tai chi can also improve balance while promoting flexibility and core strength.

A well-rounded approach that incorporates strength training, flexibility work, and balance exercises provides the best protection against sciatic pain. Consistency is key, as making these activities a regular part of a fitness routine will yield the greatest benefits over time. Additionally, focusing on proper posture, lifting techniques, and ergonomic adjustments in daily life can further support a resilient body.

By strengthening key muscle groups, maintaining flexibility, and enhancing balance, individuals can build a body that is more resistant to sciatic pain and injury. With the right combination of exercises and mindful movement, it is possible to achieve long-term spinal health and continue enjoying an active, pain-free lifestyle.

Chapter 10: Ergonomics and Lifestyle Changes

Many people unknowingly put strain on their lower back and sciatic nerve through poor posture, improper workspace setups, and unhealthy lifestyle habits. While sciatica can be caused by underlying medical conditions, everyday choices play a major role in both triggering and managing symptoms. Making small but effective adjustments can significantly reduce pain and support long-term spinal health.

This chapter goes through the key changes that can make a difference, starting with setting up an ergonomic workspace to prevent unnecessary strain. I'll also cover posture tips for daily activities, from lifting and walking to sitting correctly, ensuring that movements support rather than stress the spine. Lastly, we'll discuss the importance of maintaining a healthy weight and eating an anti-inflammatory diet to reduce pressure on the sciatic nerve and promote overall spinal well-being.

By implementing these simple yet impactful strategies, individuals can create an environment and lifestyle that support a pain-free back, making it easier to manage sciatica and prevent future flare-ups.

Ergonomics and lifestyle changes play a crucial role in both preventing and managing sciatica. Many people unknowingly put unnecessary strain on their lower back and sciatic nerve through poor posture, improper workspace setups, and unhealthy lifestyle habits. Making key adjustments in these areas can help reduce pain and support long-term spinal health.

How to set up your workspace to avoid sciatica

Setting up a workspace that promotes good posture and spinal alignment is essential for those who spend long hours sitting. A poorly arranged workstation can lead to slouching, excessive lower back pressure, and sciatic nerve irritation. To create an ergonomic setup, start by ensuring that your chair provides adequate lumbar support. Sitting with your lower back pressed against the chair's support helps maintain the spine's natural curve and prevents unnecessary strain. The chair height should allow your feet to rest flat on the floor, with your knees at a 90-degree angle. Your desk and computer monitor should be positioned so that your screen is at eye level, reducing the tendency to lean forward and strain the neck and shoulders. If possible, consider using a standing desk or alternating between sitting and standing throughout the day to alleviate prolonged pressure on the lower back.

Tips for better posture during daily activities

Maintaining proper posture during daily activities is another critical factor in reducing sciatic pain. Many everyday movements, such as lifting, walking, and even sitting, can contribute to poor spinal alignment if not done correctly. When lifting objects, always bend at the knees rather than the waist, keeping the back straight and using the legs to power the movement. Avoid twisting the spine while carrying heavy items, as this can place undue stress on the lower back. When standing, distribute weight evenly between both feet, rather than shifting to one side, which can lead to muscle imbalances and strain. Sitting for extended periods should be broken up with short walks and stretches to keep the muscles engaged and prevent stiffness. Small adjustments, such as engaging the core while sitting or standing tall with shoulders relaxed, can have a significant impact over time.

Managing weight and diet for spinal health

In addition to posture and ergonomics, managing weight and maintaining a healthy diet contribute to spinal health and sciatica prevention. Excess weight, particularly around the midsection, increases the load on the spine and can exacerbate sciatic nerve compression. Achieving and maintaining a healthy weight through balanced nutrition and regular exercise can reduce strain on the lower back and improve overall mobility. A diet rich in anti-inflammatory foods, such as leafy greens, fatty fish, nuts, and berries, can help reduce inflammation that may be contributing to sciatic pain. Staying well-hydrated is also essential, as spinal discs require proper hydration to maintain their structure and function effectively.

Making ergonomic and lifestyle changes does not require drastic alterations; even small adjustments can yield significant improvements in spinal health and overall comfort. By ensuring proper workspace setup, adopting better posture habits, and maintaining a healthy weight and diet, individuals can take proactive steps toward reducing sciatica symptoms and preventing future occurrences. Long-term success often comes from consistency, and incorporating these changes into daily routines can lead to lasting relief and improved quality of life.

Chapter 11: Long term strategies

Managing sciatica isn't just about dealing with pain when it flares up—it's about taking proactive steps to prevent it from returning. By recognising early warning signs, maintaining an active lifestyle, and managing stress effectively, individuals can significantly reduce the risk of future flare-ups and enjoy long-term spinal health.

In this chapter, I explain some of the key strategies for keeping sciatica at bay. We'll start by identifying the subtle signs that often precede a recurrence, allowing for early intervention before symptoms escalate. Next, we'll discuss the importance of staying active, highlighting exercises that strengthen the spine and prevent nerve compression. Finally, we'll examine the role of stress in pain management and how relaxation techniques can help keep both the body and mind in balance.

By incorporating these long-term habits into daily life, individuals can take control of their condition, build resilience against future episodes, and continue living an active, pain-free life.

Managing sciatica is not just about addressing pain when it arises but also about implementing long-term strategies to prevent recurrence. By recognising early warning signs, maintaining an active lifestyle, and managing stress effectively, individuals can reduce the likelihood of future flare-ups and enjoy long-term spinal health.

Recognising early warning signs of recurrence

One of the most important aspects of long-term sciatica management is recognising the early warning signs of a potential recurrence. Many people who have experienced sciatica in the past will notice subtle symptoms before a full-blown episode occurs. These may include mild lower back discomfort, occasional tingling or numbness in the leg, or a sensation of tightness in the buttocks or hamstrings. Paying attention to these signs and taking action early can prevent symptoms from worsening. Gentle stretching, adjusting posture, or temporarily reducing high-impact activities can help mitigate the issue before it becomes debilitating. Developing an awareness of personal triggers, such as prolonged sitting, improper lifting techniques, or specific activities that tend to exacerbate symptoms, allows individuals to take proactive steps in modifying their habits.

Staying active for life

Staying active is crucial for maintaining a healthy spine and preventing sciatic nerve irritation. While rest may be necessary during acute flare-ups, long-term inactivity can lead to muscle weakness, reduced flexibility, and an increased risk of recurrence. Regular exercise helps keep the muscles that support the spine strong and resilient. Low-impact activities such as swimming, walking, cycling, and yoga are excellent choices for individuals managing sciatica. Strength training that focuses on core stabilisation, glute activation, and spinal support can further reduce the likelihood of nerve compression. Consistency is key, as making exercise a regular part of a routine will yield better results than sporadic efforts. Incorporating movement into daily life—such as taking the stairs instead of the elevator, standing up and stretching every hour, or practicing good posture while sitting—can contribute to ongoing spinal health.

Stress management and its role in pain prevention

Stress management is another essential component of long-term sciatica prevention. Chronic stress can increase muscle tension, especially in the lower back and hips, which may contribute to nerve compression. Additionally, stress can heighten the brain's perception of pain, making symptoms feel more intense than they actually are. Implementing relaxation techniques such as deep breathing, mindfulness, or meditation can help regulate the body's stress response and minimise tension. Activities like yoga or tai chi not only promote flexibility and strength but also encourage relaxation and mental well-being. Prioritising adequate sleep, staying hydrated, and engaging in hobbies or activities that promote relaxation can further reduce overall stress levels.

By recognising early warning signs, committing to regular physical activity, and managing stress effectively, individuals can develop a long-term approach to sciatica prevention. These strategies not only reduce the risk of flare-ups but also promote overall spinal health and well-being. Consistently integrating these habits into daily life ensures that individuals remain in control of their condition and continue to lead an active, pain-free lifestyle.

Part 5: Resources and Support

Chapter 12: Frequently Asked Questions

Sciatica can be a confusing and frustrating condition, leaving many people searching for clear answers about its causes, treatments, and long-term management. With so much information available, it can be difficult to separate helpful advice from misinformation.

In this chapter, I'll answer some of the most frequently asked questions about sciatica, covering topics such as its causes, how long it lasts, the best treatment approaches, and when to seek medical attention. We'll also clarify common concerns about exercise, sitting, home remedies, and whether surgery is necessary for lasting relief.

By providing straightforward, evidence-based answers, this chapter aims to give individuals the knowledge they need to manage their symptoms with confidence. Whether you're experiencing sciatica for the first time or looking for ways to prevent future flare-ups, having the right information can make all the difference in your recovery and long-term spinal health.

Sciatica can be a confusing and frustrating condition, and many people have similar questions about its causes, treatment, and management. Below are some of the most frequently asked questions, along with clear and concise answers to help guide individuals toward better understanding and relief.

- **What causes sciatica?**

Sciatica is most often caused by compression or irritation of the sciatic nerve, typically due to a herniated disc, spinal stenosis, or muscle imbalances. Other causes include pregnancy, poor posture, and prolonged sitting.

- **How long does sciatica last?**

The duration of sciatica varies depending on the severity of the condition and the effectiveness of treatment. Mild cases may resolve within a few weeks, while chronic cases can persist for months or even longer.

- **Is bed rest good for sciatica?**

Prolonged bed rest is generally not recommended, as it can lead to muscle stiffness and worsening symptoms. Gentle movement, stretching, and activity modifications are typically more beneficial.

- **What exercises should I avoid with sciatica?**

High-impact exercises such as running, heavy lifting, deep squats, and exercises that involve twisting the spine should be avoided during a sciatica flare-up. Focus on low-impact movements and stretches instead.

- **Can sciatica heal on its own?**

In many cases, sciatica can improve with time and conservative treatments such as stretching, physical therapy, and lifestyle changes. However, if symptoms persist or worsen, medical intervention may be necessary.

- **When should I see a doctor?**

Seek medical attention if sciatica symptoms last longer than six weeks, significantly impact daily life, or are accompanied by severe weakness, loss of bladder or bowel control, or numbness in the saddle area.

- **Does sitting make sciatica worse?**

Sitting for long periods can put pressure on the lower back and sciatic nerve, worsening symptoms. Using an ergonomic chair, taking frequent breaks, and maintaining good posture can help alleviate discomfort.

- **Are there any effective home remedies for sciatica?**

Yes, applying heat or ice packs, gentle stretching, over-the-counter pain relievers, and using a supportive mattress can help manage symptoms at home.

- **Will losing weight help with sciatica?**

Maintaining a healthy weight reduces pressure on the spine and can decrease the likelihood of sciatic nerve compression, making it an important factor in long-term sciatica management.

- **Is surgery the only permanent solution?**

Surgery is generally considered a last resort for sciatica that does not respond to conservative treatments. Many people find lasting relief through physical therapy, exercise, and lifestyle adjustments without needing surgery.

Understanding these common concerns can help individuals navigate their sciatica journey with greater confidence. While every case is different, having clear answers to frequently asked questions can provide reassurance and direction in managing the condition effectively.

Chapter 13: Tools and Resources

Effectively managing sciatica goes beyond medical treatment and exercise—having the right tools and resources can make a significant difference in both comfort and long-term recovery. From ergonomic products that support spinal health to online communities offering guidance and encouragement, the right resources empower individuals to take control of their condition and find lasting relief.

In this chapter, I'll talk you through a few essential tools that can help alleviate sciatic pain, including ergonomic chairs, foam rollers, and massage devices. I'll also highlight the value of online support groups, where individuals can share experiences, learn from others, and stay motivated throughout their recovery journey. Finally, I'll provide recommendations for further reading and trusted sources of information for those who want to deepen their understanding of sciatica and spinal health.

By equipping yourselves with the right tools, support networks, and educational materials, you can take a proactive approach to managing their symptoms, improving mobility, and enhancing your overall well-being.

Managing sciatica effectively often requires more than just medical treatment and exercise; the right tools and resources can make a significant difference in comfort and long-term recovery. From ergonomic products to supportive communities and further reading, utilising these resources can help individuals take control of their condition and find lasting relief.

Recommended products (e.g., ergonomic chairs, foam rollers)

One of the most useful categories of tools for sciatica sufferers is ergonomic products. Sitting for long periods, especially with poor posture, can worsen symptoms by placing additional strain on the lower back and sciatic nerve. An ergonomic chair with lumbar support and adjustable features can help maintain proper spinal alignment and reduce discomfort. Similarly, standing desks provide an alternative to prolonged sitting, allowing for better posture and reduced nerve compression. For those who spend a lot of time driving, seat cushions with memory foam or gel inserts can alleviate pressure on the lower back and hips.

Foam rollers and massage tools are also valuable for relieving muscle tightness and improving flexibility. A foam roller can be used to release tension in the lower back, glutes, and hamstrings—muscles that, when tight, contribute to sciatic nerve irritation. Massage guns or tennis balls can also be used for targeted deep-tissue relief. Investing in a high-quality yoga or stretching mat can make daily mobility exercises more comfortable and effective.

As I mentioned earlier, you can scan the following QR code for a list of my recommended tools to relieve the symptoms of sciatica so you know the exact products I recommend to my patients:

Online communities and support groups

Beyond physical tools, online communities and support groups provide emotional and practical support for individuals dealing with sciatica. Connecting with others who share similar experiences can be both encouraging and educational. Online forums, such as those found on Reddit, Facebook, and dedicated health websites, allow people to exchange tips, ask questions, and share recovery stories. Many social media platforms also feature groups specifically for chronic pain sufferers, where members provide support and motivation. Additionally, some physiotherapy and chiropractic clinics offer virtual support groups, where individuals can receive professional guidance and peer encouragement.

Further reading and studies

For those who want to deepen their understanding of sciatica and spinal health, there are numerous books, articles, and studies available. Books such as "The Back Mechanic" by Dr. Stuart McGill and "Treat Your Own Back" by Robin McKenzie provide evidence-based approaches to managing back pain and sciatica. Scientific studies published in journals like Spine and The Journal of Orthopaedic & Sports Physical Therapy offer insights into the latest research on nerve pain, treatment efficacy, and rehabilitation strategies. Websites such as the National Institute of Neurological Disorders and Stroke (NINDS) and Mayo Clinic also provide reliable, research-backed information on sciatica and related conditions. I also write on various topics on my own blog; **www.aginjuryrehab.co.uk** so feel free to check that out.

Having the right tools and resources in place can make a substantial difference in managing sciatica effectively. By incorporating ergonomic solutions, utilising self-massage and stretching tools, engaging with supportive communities, and continuing to educate themselves, individuals can take a proactive role in their recovery. A well-rounded approach that combines physical, emotional, and educational support can empower individuals to manage their symptoms and improve their quality of life.

Chapter 14: When to seek help

While many cases of sciatica can be managed with self-care, exercise, and lifestyle adjustments, there are times when professional medical help is necessary. Recognising when symptoms indicate a more serious underlying condition can make all the difference in receiving the right treatment and achieving long-term relief.

In this chapter, I'll go through the red flags that require urgent medical attention, including severe pain, loss of sensation, muscle weakness, or symptoms of cauda equina syndrome. I'll also explore how to choose the right healthcare provider, from A&E and physiotherapists to chiropractors, orthopaedic specialists, and pain management experts. Understanding when and where to seek help ensures that individuals receive appropriate care, preventing complications and supporting a faster recovery.

By staying informed about when to escalate treatment, you can make confident decisions about your health and take proactive steps toward lasting sciatica relief.

While many cases of sciatica can be effectively managed with lifestyle changes, exercises, and non-surgical treatments, there are times when seeking professional help is necessary. Recognising red flags that indicate a more serious underlying condition and choosing the right healthcare provider can make a significant difference in the effectiveness of treatment and long-term recovery.

Recognising red flags that need immediate attention

One of the most critical aspects of managing sciatica is knowing when symptoms require immediate medical attention. While mild to moderate cases can often improve with self-care, certain warning signs indicate a more serious issue that should not be ignored. Sudden and severe pain that rapidly worsens, especially after an injury, may indicate nerve damage or a structural issue such as a herniated disc or spinal fracture. Loss of sensation or weakness in the leg, particularly if it affects mobility, is another warning sign that requires urgent evaluation. In rare but serious cases, sciatica can be associated with cauda equina syndrome, a condition where nerve compression in the lower spine leads to loss of bladder or bowel control, numbness in the saddle area (inner thighs and buttocks), or severe leg weakness. This is a medical emergency that requires immediate surgical intervention.

How to choose the right healthcare provider

For individuals who experience persistent sciatica symptoms lasting longer than six weeks, or if pain is interfering with daily life, consulting a healthcare provider is recommended. Choosing the right provider depends on the severity of symptoms and the preferred approach to treatment. A primary care physician can be a good starting point, as they can evaluate symptoms, provide initial treatment options, and refer to specialists if necessary. Physical therapists are excellent resources for those looking to improve mobility and reduce pain through targeted exercises and movement strategies. Chiropractors may help with spinal adjustments, particularly if misalignment is contributing to nerve compression.

For those with more severe or persistent symptoms, a specialist such as an orthopaedic surgeon or neurologist may be required. Orthopaedic specialists focus on conditions affecting the musculoskeletal system, including spinal issues, while neurologists specialise in nerve-related conditions and can assess whether sciatica is due to an underlying neurological disorder. Pain management specialists can also be valuable for individuals dealing with chronic pain, offering interventions such as corticosteroid injections or nerve blocks to alleviate discomfort.

When choosing a healthcare provider, it is important to consider factors such as experience, credentials, and treatment philosophy. Seeking providers who have experience in treating sciatica and spinal conditions ensures that they understand the best evidence-based approaches to care. Patients should also feel comfortable discussing their symptoms and treatment preferences, as open communication is key to successful recovery. Reading reviews, seeking recommendations, and verifying credentials can help ensure that individuals receive the best possible care.

Recognising when to seek professional help and choosing the right healthcare provider can prevent complications and support long-term relief from sciatica. While self-care strategies can be effective for many people, timely medical intervention can provide clarity, reassurance, and access to the most appropriate treatments. By staying informed and proactive, individuals can take control of their condition and work toward a pain-free future.

Closing thoughts…

Sciatica can be a challenging condition, but understanding its causes, treatments, and long-term management strategies empowers individuals to take control of their recovery. Throughout this book, we have explored the many facets of sciatica, from recognising symptoms and seeking professional care to adopting lifestyle changes that promote long-term spinal health. By implementing the right combination of self-care, exercise, and medical guidance, most people can find significant relief and regain their mobility.

Recap of Key Takeaways

One of the key takeaways from this book is that movement is essential for both pain relief and prevention. While rest may be necessary during acute flare-ups, prolonged inactivity often worsens symptoms. Engaging in targeted exercises, strengthening key muscle groups, and incorporating flexibility and balance training can help build a more resilient body. Ergonomics and posture play a significant role in daily comfort, and making small adjustments to workspaces, sleep positions, and lifting techniques can have a profound impact on symptom management.

Additionally, we have emphasised the importance of listening to your body and recognising when professional help is needed.

While many cases of sciatica improve with conservative treatments, severe or persistent symptoms may require intervention from healthcare providers. Understanding when to seek help and choosing the right specialist can prevent complications and lead to more effective treatment outcomes.

Next Steps

For those just beginning their journey toward recovery, the most important step is to take action. Whether it's incorporating gentle stretches into your daily routine, adjusting your workstation, or seeking advice from a medical professional, each positive step brings you closer to a pain-free life. Recovery takes time, and setbacks may occur, but persistence and consistency are key.

Most importantly, remember that you are not alone. Millions of people experience sciatica, and many have successfully managed their symptoms and regained their quality of life. Support is available through healthcare professionals, online communities, and personal networks. Stay patient, stay proactive, and trust that your efforts will lead to lasting relief.

By applying the knowledge and strategies outlined in this book, you can take control of your health and work toward a future free from sciatic pain. Keep moving forward, stay committed to your well-being, and embrace the journey to a stronger, healthier you.

Good luck!

And thanks again for supporting me buy purchasing this book.

I hope you've found it helpful in the ongoing battle against back pain and sciatica!

Arun

Printed in Dunstable, United Kingdom

64410560R00050